The Life of the CP Butterfly

The Story of Aleya's Journey

Aleya K. Linkous

Crossroads Publishing, LLC—620-204-1710
www.crossroadspublishingllc.com
ISBN: 978-1-970396-17-1
Author Aleya K. Linkous
Covert Design Idea Aleya K. Linkous
Cover Art John Wood`
Edited by Lacy Winter
Authentically Written and Designed

Special thanks to my incredible editor and manager, John Wood, without whom I couldn't have achieved this goal.

Tireless hours were spent curating the words within this book and meticulously designing the beautiful covers.

Special shout-out to my mom, Angela Cichetti-Linkous, for never giving up on me and for shaping me into the woman I am today; thank you for allowing me to achieve my goal of writing my life story.

Dedication

To my grandparents, my two angels in heaven:

Thank you for the faith, the lessons, and the memories. I hope I make you both proud. You left your love imprinted in my heart, my mind, and my soul, forever.

Preface

Starting The Journey

A couple lived in Baltimore, Maryland. They married and were ready for the gift of a child. Unfortunately, however, the wife couldn't have children. After some thought, they decided to pursue adoption. They selected a local adoption agency. On August 13, 1986, the couple, as well as both sets of grandparents, were present at Baltimore International Airport to receive their bundle of joy. I was only seven months old, having entered the world on March 18. I weighed only five pounds and was so tiny I had to wear baby doll clothes.

My adoptive mother wanted my name to be Aleya, which means precious flower in Indian culture.

My adoptive father wanted to name me Kàri. They settled on a combination of both: Aleya Karin Linkous. This is my story.

Chapter 1

Indian Butterball and New Therapies

Because I was born in India, my internal clock was on India time. This meant I slept all day and was up all night in Maryland time. My poor mom couldn't get any rest. According to her, I cried a lot because I was always hungry. The doctor had given instructions to only feed me a couple ounces of formula every couple of hours; due to the fact I was so tiny. That only lasted a few weeks. When she switched me to larger-ounce bottles, I cried less, and was a happy baby gaining weight. I became a little butterball and was thriving! My mom started to notice something was not quite right when I missed a milestone. The neighbor's baby, who was around the same age as me, would come over and was able to sit up, which was something I could not do. By then, I was between eighteen months old and two years old. We went to Johns Hopkins Children's Hospital and stayed there for about seven days while they ran a battery of tests, including brain scans and hearing tests.

By the end of the week, they told my mom I wouldn't be able to walk, talk, or comprehend like other children. They also said she should have institutionalized me from the get-go. She listened to them, but in heart, knew differently. She knew what I was capable of. It was still earth-shattering to hear as a mom. She then enrolled me in a special school:

Rolling Road School. They taught me sign language. The therapist and my mom also made sure I received speech, physical, and occupational therapy while there. Mom eventually took me out of that school because they seemed to be holding my progress back, keeping me on the same level as the other kids. As of January 2026, that school is now permanently closed.

What happened next was a miracle; I started to make sounds. When I was about two years old, my mom went to view a mobile home. The seller had cats, and they rubbed up against me while I was being held by my mom. I uttered my first sound that day.

Mom told my grandparents what had happened, and suddenly they were babysitting me while my mom drove to the pound to select a cat for us. We named her Puff, since I could make the "puh" sound.

When I was around three, my Mom-Mom would babysit me at night, while my mom worked as a bartender. Mom-Mom would give me Coca-Cola watered down with ice in my bottle, along with ice cream and other yummy stuff. Perhaps that's where my love of soda started, since my mom only gave me apple juice up until that point. My mom wasn't very happy with Mom-Mom about the soda!

Chapter 2

My First Surgery

When I was about seven, I had a hamstring release, a tendon release, and Botox injections.

We searched for the best surgeon that we could find. We found one in New Jersey.

The hamstring release would stop my toes from pointing upward, and the tendon release in my ankles was so my feet wouldn't turn in. Lastly, the Botox injections in targeted muscles were to relax certain muscle groups.

The whole surgery took between six to eight hours to complete. We only had a few visits to see the surgeon given the distance of the offices from Maryland to New Jersey. Unfortunately, I don't remember the visits that much.

We rented a white minivan so my mom, my grandparents, my stepfather, Joe, and myself could travel up to New Jersey in comfort. We left early in the morning. I remember everyone hugging me before I was wheeled back for the surgery. The next thing I remember was having the gas mask placed on my face. It smelled like the gasoline you use to fill up your car.

After the long surgery, I remember waking up with the mask still on my face, smelling like the gas pump.

In the recovery room they gave me apple juice and graham crackers. I had two white casts on my legs up to my knees. I was in the recovery room for a couple of hours. Then, it was time to head back home in the white minivan. They carefully carried me and placed me in the van. I remember being very hungry and a little sick to my stomach. On the road, they stopped at KFC and asked what I wanted. I replied, "Chicken, please." Due to the grease, they were scared to give it to me. But everyone took what they wanted and left a few pieces of yummy chicken in the bucket for me. I really enjoyed the chicken and never felt sick! My recovery was long, and I was given muscle relaxers. But I was able to climb the steps even with the casts on my legs, and I could crawl to the bathroom on my own, as well as my bedroom.

I had plenty of things to do while recuperating, such as coloring pretty pictures in coloring books, and doodling on blank drawing paper. The casts were removed after about four to six weeks, but I don't remember much of that visit, either. I was just thrilled to go back home and take a bath!

A few months after that, in the summer, I was playing in the back yard near the sand pool pad. All I remember is stepping backward and falling. A bone was sticking up in my leg and I was screaming. Mom came running out, and the neighbors called the ambulance. The paramedics explained that I had dislocated my knee. Mom asked if they could pop it back into place, but they said it would be better to take me to the emergency room, so that's what they did.

Once there, they gave me a shot to help with the pain until the doctor could put my knee back into place. While we waited, mom called my stepfather and he was there in a flash. After the doctor fixed my knee, he put it in a knee immobilizer so the knee would remain straight. The staff showed my mom how to put my knee back in place, for future reference. I was loaded up in the van and taken home. The next day, we rented a wheelchair and had fun at the science center.

Chapter 3

Walking Through Woodbridge Valley

I attended Woodbridge Valley School from second through sixth grade.

I don't remember much about my early years there, except the friends I made had a range of special needs: some with Down syndrome, some had tracheostomies, and others were in wheelchairs. A couple of them had nurses, too. We all got along pretty well, except some of them liked pulling my hair. I had a crush on a boy who was a Jehovah's Witness. I always thought it was sad that he couldn't take part in any birthday parties or holiday events. Another boy had the sweetest nurse to care for him. She rode the bus with us. That guy always had a smile on his face when I was around. He had two other sisters, and a brother at home who was adopted. He had accommodation in school since he found the coursework difficult. Unfortunately, though, his home life was made unbearable by his adoptive parents. I felt lucky to have my adoptive mom. The school was not in our district, but Mom fought for me to go there. I had an IEP which stated what special accommodations I needed to be successful in an educational setting: a note-taker, assistive technology, more time on assignments and double the amount of time for tests.

I was mainstreamed between regular and special education classes during my days in school. I really enjoyed spending most of my day on the regular side of classes. I made a lot of friends there.

I technically was held back a grade so I could stay with my friends, which was nice. I had met a lot of people who became close friends. I developed a crush on someone in the fourth grade who I was mainstreamed with. I also met my best friend.

By fifth grade I was in all regular classes. We joked it was the year from hell since the teacher was new. She did not like that I had an aid to help with my notes and schoolwork. I had an Apple AlphaSmart word processor to do some of my assignments on. The only problem was it could be hard to see what you were typing on the small, flat screen. Scrolling up to see what was written was a pain in the neck.

My mom started to argue with the technology department about getting me an actual laptop. I believe it took around two or three years to secure a Dell laptop. I was sad when fifth grade was over, but glad to have met my best friend. During that year, we discovered Puff had a tumor that took up most of her stomach, so we decided to have her put to sleep. That was a very sad time for both me and Mom. Woodbridge added on a sixth-grade building for a year. As students, we all loved it. We had two teachers: Mrs. Bogart and Ms. Jenawick. We had class cookouts at one of the state parks. We had the best time, with games like horseshoes, croquet, and other games. I remember picking up hamburger buns from McDonald's by the crate. At Christmastime we created pretty decent-sized gingerbread houses. It was my first time making them. We used graham crackers for the walls and roofs. I used ribbon candy, gum drops, and other candies to decorate mine. It was featured in the display case at the front of the school for everyone to see. I was proud of my gingerbread house decorating skills!

We had book fairs and a science fair, in which I won honorable mention for my growing crystal project.

There were only a couple of months left of school when Mrs. Bogart was offered a job in South Carolina at the aquarium. I remember taking a class picture on her

lap, crying because it was her last day, before Ms. Chase took over. As you can see, sixth grade was a blast. I had a scrapbook party at Michael's craft store for my birthday that year. A handful of friends attended. They all gave me *NSYNC gifts. It was a nice change, since I'd only had bowling birthday parties for the four years before, with close family and friends.

When I was twelve, I took a week-long vacation over the summer. My occupational therapist, who was so close to the family that I called her Aunt Nancy, joined my mom and I on the trip to Ocean City, Maryland.

We had fun at the arcade during the day, which was located on the boardwalk.

We also went back at night a few times, trying to score enough tickets to win a seal figurine I really liked, housed in the arcade's prize case.

They had a range of games there, from bowling to more adult games. We also went to the movies one rainy night to see a Disney movie; I believe it was Mulan. We shopped during the day and had lunch at restaurants like Applebee's that were located around the shopping area. It was truly a week of treasured memories.

Chapter 4

Surprises in Year Seven

I almost had major surgery the year before seventh grade. You didn't expect me to start off with that, did you? My mom got married, for the third time, to a truck driver named Joe. I wore a cream-colored dress with roses on the front. My stepfather asked her to marry him with a small, gold, heart-shaped ring. It was a really cute courthouse wedding. Another major event happened in year seven: I got a puppy named Ginger!

I wrote letters on the tablet just about every week begging for a dog. I even promised to scoop the dog poop. Well, one day, my stepfather came home from being on the road, and everyone in my immediate family discussed getting a dog. They all decided it was a good idea.

My pop-pop wanted us to get a German Shepherd since he used to raise them for the military. He also had two of his own at the current time. My mom wouldn't have that, since she'd grown up around them.

My stepfather agreed it would be nice to have a dog for protection. We went to the pound that was about an hour away from our house. I walked by all the sad puppies' eyes staring at me. One dog in particular caught my eye. She was mainly black, with brown mixed in, and a white patch on her chest. When the pound attendant came to ask what we were interested in, they told us the dog was part beagle and mutt. There were other people looking at her but they changed their minds. We got to bring her home! She'd just had her shots and deworming, so she sat in the back of the van with me. We already had a purple collar and leash ready for our new friend.

We drove along and the next thing my mom heard was the puppy throwing up, along with me. Mom had to pull over and get us cleaned up as best as she could to continue driving home. I named her Ginger due to her coloring.

She was taught how to walk beside me on a retractable leash, and to sit up and take mini-sized dog bone snacks gently from my hands. She was always with me in the backyard on my swing set which my pop-pop and uncle built for me. Once, she was a bad girl and licked the chocolate icing off a bundt cake that was left out overnight on the kitchen table for a school party the next day. I was really upset and asked my mom if Ginger was going to die. My mom called the vet. They said to watch her in case she started throwing up. Luckily, she didn't. I think she went to the bathroom outside, and it came out of that end. She was fine the next day.

Another time, she ate something in the yard that she was not supposed to. Mom walked her up the street to the vet at Westview Animal Hospital. She returned home with saddle bags of fluids to combat her reaction to whatever she had eaten in the yard. Again, she was fine after a few days.

She did have an ear mite problem that made her ears have a slight odor, and we constantly cleaned them. Because of the mites, she was not allowed upstairs where we slept. She was my best friend for twenty-three years. She came down with cancer, and it spread throughout her whole body. We did the kindest, most heartbreaking thing for her: we called around and found a vet that made home visits to put her to sleep. During the same time period, my stepfather, Joe, found a three-wheeled bike during his travels on the road. I saw him walk across the street from the church parking lot where he parked his car hauler truck. The bike was beautiful and blue. We modified the pedals by using cords over both feet, to help my feet stay on the pedals. We also put a bigger seat on it. I had a lot of fun riding up the sidewalk on it, a couple of houses one way, then back down the other way. At one point, I even decorated it for a bike contest. That was a fun time in my life.

Chapter 5

In the Middle Summer Fun

Well, guess what? You're in for a treat! That summer was the summer of concerts. We saw Brandy and Britney Spears at Merryweather Stadium, but the best of them all was *NSYNC. My mom and I searched to see where *NSYNC was playing nearby. We found out they were playing at RFC stadium in Washington, D.C. My mom was on the phone with the box office for a while.

We snagged awesome seats about seven rows back from the stage. The word 'excited' is not the right word to describe how over the moon I was about having those tickets. I talked about it nonstop for months, until finally, July 10, 2000, arrived. I woke at the crack of dawn and laid out my *NSYNC shirt and nice jeans. We got there a couple of hours early, so we had enough time to deal with parking and the actual travel to the stadium. The artist Pink opened up for them. She had a pretty cool stage performance, plus some great music. A few people were irritated because I was holding on to the rope for balance, but security was okay with it. I loved it when during part of their show they sang and danced in the middle aisle. I loved seeing Justin Timberlake!

The show was around three hours of endless screaming and fun. These are memories I will cherish forever.

Chapter 6

The Culture Shock of Southwest Academy

I attended Southwest Academy (SWA) for both seventh and eighth grade. It was a uniform-wearing school, but my mom refused to buy the uniform polo shirt from the school store, due to the steep price and safety factor. Because of this, no one knew where I attended school. I wore the same light-colored polo shirts and khaki pants to school. People would push me into the lockers when the bell rang, and I would have to leave class early so that would not occur. One of my favorite classes was art; we created a lot of really cool things there. I also enjoyed my seventh-grade science class.

The summer before entering eighth grade, our neighbor kept hearing little cries from our hedge, so Mom went to investigate. The next thing I knew, she was walking up the back deck with something in her shirt. I heard the cries of kittens. There were three kittens there with their eyes barely open, covered in stink and weeds. Mom drove to PetSmart and bought kitten milk, bottles, and a bed, and we fed them every couple of hours. We did this for about two months. We didn't name them until one morning when I went downstairs to check on them and thought one was dead. I screamed for my mom.

She took that kitten to the vet, and he needed a name in order to see the doctor. We decided to call him Weeder since we found the kittens in the weeds outside. He was there for a couple of weeks, and mom would go by the vet office to check on him. She spent a ton of money on him so we decided to keep him.

The other male kitten went to a family in Reisterstown, Maryland. The female kitty went to one of the vet technicians. They were so tiny, and at one point they could fit inside tissue boxes and the 24-pack Coca-Cola boxes as well. We were sad to see them go. Between seventh and eighth grade, I met some really good friends through art class, where we made masks, comics, and other things. One of my masks was in the Baltimore County School System art show, and I even won an award.

I also made friends in the school halls. One of them had a pretty involved case of cerebral palsy, but he was really smart. We became fast friends, even though I was in eighth grade and he was in seventh grade. We played video games and laughed at my house a lot together during the summer.

Chapter 7

The World of Western Tech

I attended Western School of Environmental Science for my freshman year of high school. I had to apply to get in, and I was accepted.

That is where I became a social butterfly. I joined many social groups, and I walked the halls with my friends. I also attended the pep rallies! It was super fun. I wanted to become a cheerleader after that. We had our seven classes split into A-days and B-days. One of my favorite classes was art, and one of my favorite projects was making a whale bowl out of clay. My mom came in to help. Our whale was one of the biggest pieces to get fired up in the kiln. Once we hit the painting stage, I selected light blue paint. I danced out of my freshman year with great memories, good grades, and wonderful friends. My tenth-grade year, however, was when the train wreck happened.

Due to the fact that the school received extra grant money for my attendance, they started to say I needed too much help, and that since I needed extra time to complete assignments at home, it couldn't be me doing the work. Teachers who I once trusted suddenly began to turn on me. I became very sad and didn't want to go to school anymore. My mom hired a lawyer so she could fight for me to still go to school there. The only issue was that I had to be out of school while they fought. Well, after a few months of sitting at home, and spending my sixteenth birthday alone, I begged my mom to let me attend the local high school. She agreed, and I finished the year at Woodlawn Senior High School.

Chapter 8

Working at the Super Fresh

The summer after my sixteenth birthday, I wanted some expensive shoes. Mom said no way. If I wanted them, I would need to get a job. Well, she started to talk to her boss, in passing, about me. He finally met me, and I explained that I was sixteen and wanted a job. Within a couple of months, in July, he offered me a job doing go-backs. I learned about the aisles quickly and interacted with customers when they needed help finding an item. I also was a greeter at the front door during the evenings, handing out the sales papers. I always had a smile on my face. My first mishap at work was when I accidentally took an empty cart outside. Unfortunately, it got away from me and hit someone's car, busting out their headlight. In tears, I panicked and told my supervisor what happened. She told me not to worry about it, and the store had insurance to cover it. For the next couple of years, I did go-backs, bagging, and greeter duties.

Once I turned eighteen, there was another opportunity for me, this time in the office. I produced sale signs of all different sizes using Microsoft Excel & PowerPoint. Someone would write down the signs needed and hang them as I made them. I did that for many years. Toward the end of the journey, I did have bad luck with a manager. She said I shouldn't be making signs because too many signs were being made and with unexplained errors, so I got the union involved.

Then my supervisor decided to make an unethical move, which was to stab me in the back. I knew what she was doing; she wanted to keep the manager on her good side. I really wanted to quit because I hated being in a toxic work environment.

After a couple of months, we found out the store was going out of business. The store closed in July of 2012. I collected unemployment for as long as I could. Unfortunately, I haven't worked since then. Let this be a lesson: don't allow others to tell you what you're capable of, SHOW THEM you're capable of anything you put your mind to.

Chapter 9

Final Highs

As a junior in high school, I took some advanced placement classes, such as marketing and forensics. I tried to take a different science class to begin with, but it was short-lived. The teacher loved the outdoors WAY too much. One day he brought a bag to class, and of course, it was my luck to be sitting inches away from the bag. Well, out of the bag, he pulled a huge black snake! I jumped out of my seat so fast it made the desk move. He kept talking about it, as my classmates laughed at me. By that time, I was on the steps, headed back upstairs. I was done for the day. My mom knew something was wrong when she picked me up that afternoon. I was in tears. My mom called the teacher that evening and said I wouldn't be returning to that class until the snake was GONE.

The teacher said he was going to keep it for a couple of days since the other students liked it. I recall my mom firing back with, "She liked your class, but she will be leaving and switching to a different class!"

The teacher said that was a shame because he liked having me in class. The next morning, I went to the office and inquired about a different AP science class. Much to my surprise, they had one more spot available in forensics. I was teamed up with three other students and was the fourth added to that team.

We did a lot of projects dealing with DNA, and I really enjoyed lifting prints. We left store-bought pig's feet outside until they were covered in maggots.

I will admit, I don't know how my stomach handled looking at them. But the team members each did their part. My part was to type the report and hand it in.

I walked away from that class with a high 'B' grade and a better overview of how the forensics process works. It was, overall, a very interesting experience.

Marketing was my second favorite class, since we were learning how to write business plans for our potential businesses. Mine was a pet-sitting business, and I went to many rubber-chicken dinners for awards in marketing.

I never missed school, only once, due to having my wisdom teeth removed. My mom took a Friday off so I could have it done. I was so nervous about being put under that I hyperventilated in the chair.

They told my mom we might have to come back. She told them, "I took the day off to have this done." I settled down and said I would have it done as long as they did not put me under. The oral surgeon agreed to just numb me and put me in the twilight zone. My mom thought they were a bit crazy. After all the nervousness, I did wonderfully and went shopping that afternoon. Unfortunately, I did have a dry socket, so we had to go into the office daily for them to repack it with stuff that tasted like cinnamon. We did that for a week and I was fine.

At that point, junior year was almost over. There was a little kitty that kept crossing the street while coming to our porch for food. My mom said if she crossed the street one more time safely, then God wanted her to be our kitty. She was really sweet and friendly. We named her Missy when we had her spayed at the vet. She always had this little 'pissy' attitude on her face. She loved to cuddle and be petted.

We had her for about ten years before she became ill. We put in a feeding tube to help

with dehydration, but her little body gave up and she had to be put to sleep. It was a sad thing to see.

I finally entered my senior year with mixed emotions because I really wanted to graduate with my friends at Western Tech.

I did work-study, so I went to school until eleven a.m. every day, then went home. On Fridays, though, I had to go to work after class. I did homework on the days I left school early. It was an easy work process for me, since I had already worked a job that dealt with marketing at Super Fresh. One of many highlights of the year was being awarded a scholarship from a private organization outside of school. We had to write an essay about a word which described us and how we showed up in school. My word was 'courage'.

I wrote about a number of ways I showed up with courage. I showed up by going to a dangerous school and not getting caught up in the gangs and culture of the school (except my words!) I also showed courage through always being comfortable with my decisions and knowing what I wanted to do in the future. I remember photographers taking pictures of me as I was walking down the hall. I thought it was for the yearbook or something, but it turned out it was because I was one of the winners of the scholarship!

I had decided not to go to prom at first, but everyone said I might regret it. One of the guys I worked with volunteered to take me as friends. I went to the India store and found a pretty dress. It was a long night of dancing and an afterparty. I was, and still am, glad I went. I also was inducted into the National Honor Society. I finished in the top ten percent of my class in 2005. One of my favorite parts of graduation was senior pictures. I had my own little photoshoot at the studio. I wanted to model back then, so it was a good start.

On graduation day I wore a black spaghetti-strap dress that had flowers on it. We had to use bobby pins to secure the hat to my head, since it was too big.

I had mixed emotions about walking across the stage. I wanted to graduate from somewhere else. I did receive a standing ovation, which felt really good.

It also helped that I had proven my doubters wrong. Not only did I finish high school, but I finished in the top percentage!

Chapter 10

The Start of Catonsville Community College of Baltimore County

Upon starting college, I was required to take placement tests. I took two English tests and one reading test. In addition, I signed up for remedial math classes.

My first few semesters consisted of taking those pass/fail courses. The reading and writing courses were good refreshers. I was involved with the Student Government Association for the school, and also active in the Bible club. I took some health and stress management classes, too.

The teacher was very knowledgeable and gave me pep talks when I needed them. I took art classes and wrote a paper on the blue hippo's connection to fertility for The Walters Art Museum in Baltimore. I also took an American History class and enjoyed learning the country's history. One of my favorite projects while there was my Cherokee Indian scrapbook. During that project, I met a very special note-taker named Mim. She helped me with notes, writing for tests, and proofreading papers I wrote. I took a handful of psychology classes as well since I wanted to become a school counselor. They were interesting and I learned a lot. A fun outing was going to Baltimore/Washington International Airport to welcome our troops home.

I helped my then boyfriend with OSHA certification classes since he was helping me with surgeries. I have seven more classes left to earn a degree.

Chapter 11

Major Surgeries and Relationship

In the winter of 2007, my back started to really hurt. It hurt so much that I couldn't walk up the stairs to use the bathroom, so I crawled up the stairs to my mom's room, where she was lounging on the new mattress we had recently purchased. I told her how much I was hurting, and she offered to take me to the ER for muscle relaxer shots. I turned her offer down and took some over-the-counter medication instead.

The next morning, I researched pain doctors and orthopedic doctors. The first doctor was connected to Sinai Hospital in Baltimore. She showed us my deteriorating spine using the x-rays on the wall behind me during my exam. She concluded I had scoliosis with a ten-percent curve which would only continue to worsen. She also said I needed major surgery if I wanted to walk in ten years. She didn't speak to me directly, which was very unsettling. I was twenty years old at the time, and to have her ask my mom if she had any questions, instead of asking me, felt a bit disrespectful. She also suggested that I have both legs operated on at the same time. I remember thinking to myself, "Definitely not!" We took the information she provided us with and headed home to think things over. It was kind of shocking when I sat down and told my grandparents about the visit.

Everyone thought we needed a second opinion, confirming our thoughts. We continued to do research and found Dr. A from Mt. Airy, but he saw patients at Kernan Rehabilitation Hospital. It was only about thirty minutes away from us at the time, so we went there for an appointment. He did more x-rays and watched me walk around the office. He asked why I didn't have that type of surgery when I was a teen. My mom explained that she did not want me to have to repeat surgeries as I grew. She also said she wanted me, personally, to make all the choices regarding the surgeries when I was of age.

At first, the doctor wanted to do surgery on the more-afflicted leg first, but after more thought, he chose to hold off, instead casting it and doing Botox injections as a first step.

Back at school, I met a nice guy who was completing work-study hours. We became friends, but it quickly turned into a boyfriend/girlfriend relationship. We had an age difference of twenty years between us, and my mom did not like 'C' at first, due to the large gap. He brought me a stuffed rabbit and a get-well balloon when I had the Botox and casting done on my left leg. He was a painter, and we had a disagreement with my mom about what color to paint my bedroom. We decided on a light peach color, something cheery, as I would be spending a lot of time in my room recovering from surgeries.

C and I made a lot of Blockbuster trips for movies every week, and we took trips to Ocean City, Maryland, and Busch Gardens to enjoy Water Country. Things were nice, but he was not big on kisses, cuddles, and definitely not intimacy. When his mother passed away, we got engaged, but for all the wrong reasons. I enjoyed all the fun we had, and still do to this day. I learned a lot from my relationship with C. I learned that having material things does not equal love, and that you can't stay with someone just because your family likes them. Around the same time, the neighborhood cat from the apartments across the street started to come around our side of the street. His owners had moved away and took the dog, but left him behind. His name was Nike. He had his pick of four or five porches to choose from every night, and we all made sure he was cared for. During the winter, Mom would open the door, and he would come in from the cold and snow, but at night he always wanted to go back out.

During warmer weather, all mom had to do was whistle and he would come home for dinner. Mom even got him to walk beside her, like a dog. He loved my mom, even though she chased him away with water when there was a rooster over at the playground.

Nike was around for a long time. He loved Mom so much that he waited until Mom was home before he passed away, held in her arms.

Back to the casting procedure, I felt fine until the Botox started to relax my muscles. We discovered the cast was too tight and dug into the skin on top of my foot. We called the doctor, and despite the discomfort, he insisted the cast would have to stay on. My mom hated seeing me so uncomfortable, so next thing I knew, I was seated in the bathroom in the tub on a milk crate, while she tried sawing the cast off with a small hand saw. Finally, she used a small blow torch and burnt through the cast. I was really scared. When we finally managed to remove the cast, there was a gaping hole on top of my foot. We took pictures and showed Dr. A. He had no comment, seemingly shocked into silence. When I went out, I had to wear a slipper on that foot and a regular shoe on my right foot. The next step was surgery, where the team basically broke my leg hip in order to reposition both in the right place. They also put my knee back where it belonged, did ankle transfers, cut my Achilles tendon, and lastly, cut through a lot of nerves in my foot. It was a long surgery, around six-to-eight hours. For pain management, I had a morphine pump which sent the medicine through an epidural in my back. I also had a catheter for 48 hours. The first night was a little hard to get through, but my boyfriend, C, stayed the night until I transferred to the children's hospital. They tried to help me stand the next day but I got dizzy. I had physical therapy, though, and became a little testy toward the therapists since it hurt to do what they were asking. I was there for four days before getting transferred to Mount Washington Children's Hospital to start rehab. It was embarrassing to be there, following rules geared toward children, and having a child as a roommate. But the rehab was great, and I enjoyed my stay there for the two weeks until Mom signed me out to go home. After she had signed me out, I went to eat with C and we stopped at Hollywood Video to get movies and video games. I got dizzy while there, and the staff brought me a chair to rest in.

I started outpatient physical therapy the next week. I was familiar with the therapist since I worked with him prior to the surgery. He put my foot in neutral to see how far it would go, and I cried out in pain. I attended PT three days a week at that point. After the cast came off, about six weeks later, I was put right into AFOs to hold the position of the work that Dr A had done in surgery. I had to wear shoes to bed while the brace was on. I was in physical therapy for months. About a year later, I had the same exact surgery on the right leg. The only difference was that I stayed at Kernan Hospital, instead of being transferred to Mount Washington Children's for rehabilitation. When I woke up, the pain seemed different. I got really sick from the morphine in the pain pump. I found myself pushing the button for pain relief more often. I kept telling the people around me that I would be back on the operating table in a few months. They thought I was crazy, but I knew something felt off. I stayed there for about a week doing physical therapy with the hospital team. I started outpatient therapy as soon as I got out of the hospital, with the same outpatient therapists I had before, about three times a week. I got the cast off, and at my request, they took follow-up x-rays of my right hip where the hardware was located. Nothing was visibly out of place, but I could not deny the pain. Dr. A said I needed to let it heal for about six months. After six months, he decided to reopen the hardware site. When he moved the hardware out of the way, pus started to seep from the area. I had an infection hiding behind the hardware! He cleared up the infection site and removed the hardware with a quick surgery. Everything hurt more, but I got through it, and to this day I consider that experience a reminder of how resilient I am to the never-ending challenges I have faced.

Chapter 12

Moving Up and Meeting E

I met E in a disabled chat room and we quickly became friends. We talked for about seven months before finally meeting in person at my job. After Super Fresh closed, I took a few trips to Pennsylvania to check out things while collecting unemployment and to spend time with E. By 2015, I packed my bags and moved to Pennsylvania with E, where I stayed for seven years. There, we added a black kitty named Lotus to our family. I would say we picked Lotus from the shelter, but she really picked us. We sat in a room with all the cats and waited to see which one came to us. E noticed Lotus Marie hiding behind another cat, and he said hi. Next thing I remember, Lotus had climbed onto E's lap, and then mine, enjoying the attention. She must have known she was going home with us, because she sat right on top of the carrier, waiting to leave! I think we surprised everyone by adopting a black cat on Halloween, but it worked out perfectly. We had a great Thanksgiving and Christmas that year, plus a very fun party on New Year's Eve, with E's coworker who was in a band, and his family. During the seven years in Pennsylvania, we got two more cats: Vivian and Samual. Vivian was from the same shelter where we had adopted Lotus. She was a mommy's girl at first, then became a daddy's girl. We only had her for six months before she became ill and passed away. Samual was given to us by E's older son. He was definitely a mommy's boy.

Unfortunately, he ran out the door one day, never to be seen again. E and I had a good relationship. We had our ups and downs, like every couple, but we had our fun as well.

I became really independent doing paperwork, banking, and running the household alongside E. I continued physical therapy at Good Shepherd Rehab Hospital as an outpatient.

I had an awesome therapist for my mental health needs. We clicked from day one. When E worked, I had a number one protector to watch over me and the house: our dog, Cassidy.

I enjoyed holding her leash while sitting on the porch. She became very protective of us, probably overprotective. She had a little trouble with biting occasionally, but Cassidy was only trying to protect us. Around late 2020, I started to notice changes in E. He would forget where we were going for doctor's appointments and forget what day or time it was. I thought it might have been mental fog from the lockdown restrictions, as it seemed like everybody's mental health was taking a collective hit with all the fast changes in the world. By 2021, the forgetfulness became more severe, and E would forget what days he worked and the medications he took daily. In November 2021, I remember laying on the floor for a week, alone, with hardly any food or drink. I had fallen while cleaning, and E hadn't realized I was upstairs at all that week to help me off the floor. Mom knew something wasn't right, so she drove three hours to our home to check on us. She saw me lying by the door and wondered where E was. The fire department was called to help me to the car since I was so weak. They also requested an ambulance for E. That was the end of our living together. The next weekend we picked up Lotus from the local shelter to bring her back to Maryland to live with me. Animal control had picked up two of our three pets at our home. We stopped to see E at the hospital. That was the last time I felt that we were a couple. Over the next couple of months, we saw each other one last time, and he was placed in a nursing home, with many problems. Sadly, we never got to say goodbye in person.

Chapter 13

My Faith and Losing Mom-Mom

From an early age, I've always had strong faith. I found security in knowing it was God's will to have the family I was blessed with, and comfort in knowing that God made me in His image.

My family, especially my pop-pop, thought that I was reincarnated as his sister, but with many different abilities. Mom-Mom and Pop-Pop had a daughter that did not live very long, as she was born with all her organs outside of her body. Perhaps I was part of them, but given a second chance in life?

I started praying as early as I can remember, maybe between the ages of five and seven, on my best days and not-so-good ones. I really liked cross necklaces and felt extra protected by God when wearing them.

People question how and why I trust the Lord so much since I have Cerebral Palsy. My answer is simple: He gives me strength and wisdom to carry on. When I was about twelve years old, I started taking classes in preparation for my first Holy Communion. The classes were very spiritually rewarding, and I learned a lot about the Catholic faith.

I liked making my placeholder, the Lamb of God, to put over the pew so my family knew where to sit. My stepfather joked with me that I must be getting married in such a beautiful white dress. I have always expressed my faith by telling others about it. Others have invited my family to their churches for various healing ceremonies. Some of them got a little out of hand, especially when they started talking in tongues. The truth is, I do not want to be completely healed. I know, deep within me, that God created me this way for a purpose. We all have purposes in this world when we are born into it.

It takes time to identify what our purpose is in life. But we have people to look after, and issues to be involved with, before God calls us home. The Ten Commandments may offer us a little window into why someone is here so long. The Ten Commandments can also be used as guidance for what we should and shouldn’t do daily.

As I entered different stages of life, my prayers changed, too, but were always centered around God's will.

I started to attend an Episcopal church since I really enjoyed Mother Carol's sermons. They really spoke to my heart. You don't need to go to church to be a believer because God is everywhere. He is always beside us guiding us to do His Will. When a relative is ill, we wonder why they must suffer or they choose to hide their suffering from us, in an effort to protect us and not be a burden. My world fell apart in March of 2009, when Pop-Pop passed away from brain tumors.

I felt a deep sadness within my heart the day he passed into his heavenly home. I prayed a lot during that time for those who loved him. I worried about Mom-Mom the most since she lost her soulmate. I knew God would see her through it, although I couldn't help but wonder how long she would have left with us. She broke her hip sometime in 2013, but she made a complete recovery after being at a Catholic nursing home for a couple of months. She had problems with fluid buildup on her heart, and I prayed extra hard each time it occurred, hoping they could drain it off. In 2015, she was in hospice care due to her lungs and heart filling with fluid. Cognitive changes were happening, and everything seemed to keep going downhill.

On May 5, my mom called my then boyfriend, E, to ask if he was home. Then she texted me that Mom-Mom was gone. My whole body went numb, and I couldn't speak or type for a while. Eventually, when I regained some movement in my fingers, I typed OK to my mom.

I needed God so much at that moment. To top it off, I had a doctor's appointment to attend, and I literally crawled up the steps and got myself ready somehow. Lotus, my little black shelter kitty was upstairs. I began to cuddle her for comfort. Cassidy, my boyfriend's German Shepherd, was laying on the bed with Lotus, so I gave her some pets as well. To be honest, the appointment and whatever else we did that day left a big blank in my mind.

By that night, the shock finally started to settle. I noticed that I had somehow accidentally scratched E's arm from being in so much shock.

The arrangements were made, and my mom even said we did not have to travel down there from Pennsylvania, but E knew how much Mom-Mom meant to me so he gathered the money and took us down for three days of services. I did okay the first time I saw her in the casket, since I honestly did not recognize her. I sang the hymns she had selected for her service, such as "Amazing Grace." Singing the songs made me feel closer to God. Also, hearing Reverend Metcalf speak made my heart feel closer to God. My uncle Dominic was a crying mess because his mom was everything to him. People made comments about me crying so much throughout the three days, and I recall hearing people say unkind things such as, "Why does Kari have to be such a drama queen at these kinds of events?" But back to having faith, one of the events that changed my faith completely was the unexpected adoption of my son.

Chapter 14

The Joys of Pregnancy

For Valentine's Day of 2016, E and I went to the local I-Hop for a nice breakfast. When we tried to pay, we found out the man at the table behind us had paid for our meals. My body started to feel odd after Valentine's Day. I used the bathroom more, had tender spots, and was moody.

I knew deep down that I was pregnant. I messaged my family doctor and explained my symptoms to her. She referred me to an OB/GYN. I had to fill out a lot of paperwork before I could be seen. I also had to pee in a cup. When I finally got to see the doctor, I demanded a blood pregnancy test. We felt home tests were unreliable and wanted a trustworthy answer. The day before my thirtieth birthday, the office called with positive test results. E was at work, so I took a picture of myself, smiling ear-to-ear, and texted it to him. He knew right away by my smile. At my first appointment, they gave me books about baby development and changes to my diet, listened to the heartbeat, took my blood pressure and measured my belly, and even talked about E's medical history, as well as my own.

My favorite appointments were the ultrasound ones where you could see the baby inside the belly. I had about four of them. The appointments were every eight weeks at first. My craving was for Cici's pizza early on. I hated chocolate and onions almost instantly. In the early visits, they suggested an in-home nurse. I was not interested at first, due to the condition of our home and our overprotective dog. But E convinced me it was a good idea, so she came with a binder of information every couple of weeks. It helped me to see where my strong and weak points were concerning childcare. I went to a maternal medicine doctor for an extra ultrasound to check if the baby had any physical defects and to see if I needed any further pre-genetic testing. They said I did not, and that the baby looked good. Around fifteen weeks we had the gender ultrasound and found out it was a boy. I was a little disappointed but was glad he was healthy. The gestational diabetes test that occurred twice was hard to do, but I passed both times. I had the worst heartburn ever, so I took liquid medicine for it. Near the end of my pregnancy, we had visits every week in the form of childbirth classes. When I was 36 weeks, I felt him moving around a lot, so I went to my last appointment and they checked his heartbeat. His heartbeat was fine, but my blood pressure was high, so they sent me to the hospital. I had a case of mild preeclampsia, so they wanted him out as soon as possible. He was in the right position, but turned at the last minute, which meant I needed a c-section. It was scary having an epidural in my back again, but they got it on the first try. They let my partner go back with me after they placed the epidural. I was still scared but calm. They got our baby out pretty fast. I fell even more in love with him when holding him for the first time and I kissed his little head.

My partner had to stay with me at all times. I tried to breastfeed, but it did not work, so we went to bottles. The nurses lost patience with me, but I was a new mom. I enjoyed the late nights with us as a family. Every time he cried, I woke up, no matter what time it was.

He definitely had a good pair of lungs on him when it came time to eat or change his diaper!

Chapter 15

The Joys and Heartbreaks of Motherhood

I was instantly in love with our baby. When he was born, he weighed only four pounds, which is pretty small. He also had trouble keeping his body temperature regulated. The next day, the hospital's Children and Youth Services representative paid a visit to my hospital room and said they had concerns about me handling the care of my son on my own. They would feel safer if I had someone with me around the clock to help. They said it wouldn't be an issue if E didn't have to work three days a week and we had family support nearby. The other issue was the condition of our home, as they would not let the baby go home with the house as it was. For these reasons, I stayed in the hospital for seven days after my C-section, waiting for my mom to come pick up Cain and I from the hospital in Allentown, Pennsylvania. I just wanted to keep my little family together. The social workers made it seem as though they already had a foster family ready for him, but neither me nor E was about to sign over the rights for our baby to the state. Mom finally made it to the hospital and settled me and Cain in for the long ride back to Maryland. It was hard with a newborn baby, but we did it. Cain and I slept in the little spare room. I enjoyed holding him and feeding him. My mom took a week off from work to help us out. We made a post on Facebook about our situation, sharing that we were in need of help so my mom could return to work. Despite the helping hands provided by family, it was still very hard to wake up all hours of the night for feeding and diaper changes, especially for my mom, who would have to work the next day. I was really missing E and our pets back home. I also experienced a bit of postpartum depression. I knew my child needed to come first. Mom offered the suggestion of visiting the local adoption agency to learn about their process. I kept praying and asking God why He would give me the blessing of a baby, something I always wanted, if I would need all of this help to raise him.

The next day, we drove to the adoption agency. They gushed over how cute Cain was. They handed us books of possible people who wanted to adopt. I had about four families to pick from. The family I selected had a farm, and the dad was a disability lawyer. Their video spoke to my heart. Through tears, I signed all the paperwork to start the adoption process. It was close to Thanksgiving.

I went back to Pennsylvania a complete mess, but I was glad, too, in a way. I was ready to be back with E and the fur babies so we could grieve together.

I blamed myself, E, and my mom for that adoption. I blamed God for giving me my rainbow baby and then ripping him from my arms and heart.

Chapter 16

The Aftermath of Post-Adoption

Mom met the adoptive family soon after I was back in Pennsylvania. I was too busy grieving to join her, and it felt like a movie with a sad ending. I kept asking, "Why?" in between the tears. I felt numb, just pretending I could do life. Every time I saw a baby or child, tears ran down my face. I had to find a new OB/GYN doctor to look at my incision and ensure I was healing properly. I went to my primary care doctor after that to restart my medications and talk about my depression. The office personnel asked where the baby was. I couldn't speak for a few minutes, but E explained we had placed the baby with an adoptive family. After the necessary appointments, I just wanted to hide in the house, curled up with the two cats and dog. The adoption agency called to check on us and set up our Child Connect account so we could receive letters and pictures of the baby.

I wrote all the letters back and forth to the family, with little input from E. Thc pictures were hard to look at but were very cute at the same time. Christmas came and went but I didn't even care. I had been looking forward to the baby's first holiday.

Mom did send him gifts for his first Christmas, which made me feel a little bit better. Me and Mom were not on the best of terms at that time, but we were still texting each other. I forgot she was grieving as well. I thought she was just glad to have me and the baby gone from her house, but she was heartbroken as well. She offered for me to stay at her house, which was nice, but I just wanted to be with my fur babies and E. Plus, she was renting my room out. I cherished each picture and letter I received from the baby's new family. We actually have baby pictures of Finn (they renamed him Finn) and me that have the same side profile. He is definitely my twin, even as he gets older.

We now get pictures, cards, and videos, and we send gifts on his birthday, Christmas and Easter.

Chapter 17

The Gift of My Grandparents

From day one, I was very close to my mother's parents: Mom-Mom and Pop-Pop. They were always there for us, as far back as I can remember. Me and Mom-Mom had shopping days every month. We tried to get Pop-Pop to come sometimes, but we had no luck. I believe Pop-Pop tried to take me shopping once, without telling me I could have only one or two things. Me being little, I just put all sorts of things in the cart. When it was time to go, he actually bought all of the stuff I had thrown in the cart! Mom-Mom and I had a flat tire a few times and had to call Pop-Pop, but he didn't believe us. He thought we wanted him to come have lunch so he would get stuck with the bill.

When I was at Rolling Road School, I would go to McDonald's with Pop-Pop and get treated to a nice, yummy milkshake. I never liked them until I tried a taste of Pop-Pop's after doing good in occupational therapy with Miss Celia. I went to the zoo when I was quite young with my mom, Mom-Mom & Pop-Pop. I would look at the polar bears and hippos with Pop-Pop holding me. I was always a pasta girl. That's where I got the name of my little Italian Indian doll from. The first time they put a steamed crab down in front of me, I was scared. But if you put an army-sized bowl of spaghetti in front of me, I would go to town on it.

When I was about four years old, we started playing all-night bingo at the fire hall. I would sleep under the table in my Barney sleeping bag when I got tired. I got spoiled with good food and snacks all night. It was me, Mom, Mom-Mom and other guests sometimes, like Aunt Nancy and Mom-Mom's friends. I liked the bingo dotters and would sometimes try to play. Everyone had their little good luck charms with them. It was a fun time and I cherish those memories. We would visit Mom-Mom and Pop-Pop on Sundays for family dinners with the whole family there. They always had German Shepherd dogs that had to go to the basement when company came over, due to their size. The biggest, named Surge, would let people in but didn't let people leave. The sizes of both dogs were intimidating since I was so small. Every time we went there, we would call first to let them know we were coming. Their house was between thirty minutes and an hour away from our house. A lot of family members attended the family meals, such as my great-grandmother, cousins, aunts, and uncles. I was the youngest granddaughter at the time. Mom-Mom was the animal whisperer, with all the creatures visiting her on her porch every morning. She even had squirrels taking peanuts out of her hand! Chipmunks found safety under the dirt steps of her home. I used to feed the geese and ducks that would come onto their property. I always sat on Pop-Pop's lap before or after dinner.

Sometimes I sat on my cousin's lap, other times even Mom-Mom's lap, but Pop-Pop's lap was my favorite. The food was usually Italian, and dinners would get really loud with everyone there. The holidays were no different. I had two Christmases each year; one at Mom-Mom and Pop-Pop's house, and one at my house. We always rang in the new year together as a family. Shrimp macaroni salad was found at every holiday meal, along with Italian dishes, and even different meats, with all the fixings.

Every Thursday, my mom, grandparents, and a few neighbors would bowl together in a bowling league. I looked forward to having time off from school on Thursdays so I could hang out with my grandparents. The snack bar had the best food ever! I even had my own bowling balls, so I could join in the fun. My grandparents loved to eat at buffets. I started to like buffets too, because you could choose your own food. Pop-Pop and I loved the soft serve ice cream.

When I was about twelve years old, my grandparents got MSN dial-up internet service so they could play my favorite game with me, backgammon. Pop-Pop disagreed about having the internet, but Mom-Mom liked the idea of being able to communicate with me and play games with people around the world. Pop-Pop adjusted to having the internet. As I got older, we found the Pogo.com website, where we played to win the badges of the week. We chatted there, too. Those were simpler days and gave me lots of cherished memories to look back on.

When my great-grandmother passed away, the viewings in her honor were very nice. I was only ten or eleven at the time, and relatives tried to treat me as though I was clueless to what a hug was. It was upsetting, but thankfully Mom-Mom stopped it from escalating into a fight. When Mom-Mom got her inheritance money, she took me to Gardner Furniture just to look around. Well as luck would have it, I found a bedroom set that I fell in love with. I just hugged Mom-Mom and the next thing I knew she disappeared to the back of the store. By the time I found her, she had a pink slip of paper in her hand and said she bought me the bedroom set. It was going to be delivered when I was on Christmas break from school, at this point my mom and Pop-Pop had no clue what just happened. I kept asking if Mom-Mom was okay with what she just did. Also, if Pop-Pop and my mom would be okay with it. She said it was fine and we would deal with the others.

When I was about fifteen or sixteen, my grandparents decided to sell their old, run-down house. It needed so much work, plus the dogs had passed on. I had finally become close to Surge, though he was very old and couldn't get around very fast. I actually hugged and gave him some loving pets, which really surprised

Pop-Pop. I was very sad when Pop-Pop called to tell me Surge had passed on. I even offered to give Pop-Pop my dog, Ginger. By the time they sold their house to move closer to us, they had no pets. One day, Mom-Mom saw a wild cat and her kittens creep up to the door for food, and being the animal lover she was, she fed them. We called Friends of Animals to trap the mother and have her spayed. Sadly, the mother cat didn't make it through the spay surgery. Mom-Mom felt horrible and decided to keep one of the kittens, naming him Buster. I never knew that Pop-Pop even liked cats. Another time, a little calico cat appeared on my grandparents' porch, looking for food and love. Mom-Mom noticed she had no front claws and no collar on her. She called us over to meet her, and we all named her Susie. Instantly, I fell in love with her cuteness and sweetness. After Mom-Mom passed on, Mom took Susie over to her house, where she lived happily for the next ten years. She was around twenty years old when she passed, in May of 2025.

Both of my grandparents took me to Catonsville College Baltimore County and picked me up on many occasions. We usually did things such as driving to see Christmas lights, having a nice meal afterward. We discovered Pop-Pop had multiple brain tumors in early 2009. They did surgery, but it was too late. He passed away in March of 2009. The viewings took place over a long two days. It was standing room only for most of the viewings. Pop-Pop had a lot of friends! A man came up to me during the viewings and asked if I was Kari. When I told him yes, he said Pop-Pop always talked about me at the dinners they had, and I was the light of Pop-Pop's life. Mom-Mom was never the same after he passed on. She would take me to doctor's appointments or go shopping once in a while, but you could tell she missed her soulmate.

Chapter 18

Adjusting to Familiar Surroundings

I was glad to be in a safe, warm house after my week on the floor with hardly any food or drink. I was concerned about getting my belongings from E's house. At that point in time, I really thought he would get out of the hospital, and we would be back together. Unfortunately, that's not what happened. My legs were weak for a while, and I had to get used to my mom having a roommate. It definitely created some tension in the environment.

By May, everything was decided for E. The shock I felt was mind-numbing, and it felt like my metaphorical glass heart had shattered into a million pieces inside me. By October, it felt like my brain was completely shut down. I made the decision to check myself into Shepherd Pratt Hospital so they could adjust my medications and figure out why I lost my memory. I stayed there for around a month, but they couldn't find anything wrong with me. They adjusted my medications, though, which seemed to help. The doctors were concerned about sending me home due to my mobility issues, suggesting placing me in a nursing home as a temporary solution, but luckily they found a home-health organization to assist with my care. They also enlisted a "pep team," which consisted of encouraging people who came to the house weekly and monthly to make sure I was on the right medications. A case worker, nurse, and doctor came as well. I had the home health team for about six months but had the pep team until August of 2025. During the last four months of 2024, I felt more like myself. Physical therapists came from the same healthcare company twice a week until the first of January 2025.

This was a huge adjustment period for me, and one which I did NOT get accustomed to quickly. This part of my journey sticks with me all these years later because, even though it was difficult, it showed my tremendous strength and courage.

Chapter 19

Moving Along

The year of 2024 was filled with home-based physical therapy and many visits with the pep team. Though I had an entire team of people constantly coming by, I was still having issues recalling some memories. I also had some horrible nightmares when I could finally rest. Due to the lack of sleep, I began to think bugs were crawling on me. They adjusted my meds and gave me one to help me sleep. The last four months of that year were better. I felt back to my old self.

We had wonderful holidays. I really benefited from my awesome pep team, plus the great physical therapy.

Chapter 20

Turning the Page to Major Blessings

I was not reinstated for physical therapy because I needed a break. By Easter, my cat, Susie, was acting really needy and odd. She would only eat the lick able chicken treats, which I had initially received in a box of goodies for the cats. By Memorial Day, Mom called to take her to the vet. The next day she was having trouble breathing, so Mom wrapped her up in a towel, and off to the emergency vet they went. The vet said she was at least twenty years old. They told Mom she still had a heartbeat, but by the time they handed her back to my mom, she was gone. We had her cremated so she would always be with us.

By June, we began to discuss moving more seriously. We had already started getting rid of stuff we didn't need throughout the year, anyway.

By July, Mom's little junk car was in its last days, so she purchased a 2016 Nissan. It was a blessing to have found it for such a great price. Meanwhile we had our realtor evaluate our house and determine what possible repairs were needed, pricing, and take photos for the website. By early August, the house was on the market, and we started to pack. Mom looked at a couple of new places.

One of the places wouldn't allow her to look because I was not in the right age range. It was disappointing, but I knew that God would lead us to where we were supposed to be. The other 55-and-up community had a couple places available for sale, and they said as long as the homeowner was 55 or over the other people didn't need to be. There was a house back on the market after some interested people had backed out of the contract, so Mom took a look, immediately falling in love with the sun porch and layout of the house. She and the realtor placed it under contract. We really started to pack and get rid of things from that point on.

We had a handful of people interested in our former house. One of them put a contract on it. So, on August 29, the movers arrived, bright and early, to move us. The truck was overflowing with our belongings.

We arrived around 2:00 p.m. with the cats in tow. It was my first time seeing our new home. We kept the cats out on the sun porch while the movers brought everything in, placing our boxes and furniture in different areas of the house.

I was excited to have my own room and bathroom! We spent the next few months painstakingly arranging each room until things looked just how we wanted. We had a nice Thanksgiving. December was fun, and we decorated outside for Christmas with inflatables of all kinds.

We even entered the community decoration contest. We didn't win, but everyone said our house made people smile.

For Christmas, we also decorated a six-foot-tall white tree with all kinds of special ornaments. The cats did fine with the tree until the last couple of days before Christmas. They were running around, playing, when one of the top ornaments fell down and busted on the floor. It was a glass snowman, and shards went everywhere. I think it was Mocha's fault because she wouldn't look at us after it happened.

Mocha is an eleven-year-old tortoiseshell that Mom rescued back in 2014. Some neighborhood kids were hitting her with a broom. She was in heat, and Mom took her to get fixed and microchipped. It took Mocha a while to trust my mom, but in the end, it was all worth it.

Chapter 21

The Wonders of 2026

I decided this year I will try to get my faith back to where it was and lean on the Lord much more. I must say it's working pretty good so far but I'm praying for others facing major battles, not myself. I have always wanted to write a book about my life but knew I would need a good editor and manager. I have found that in John Wood, a good friend of mine who also happens to be an author himself.

This book could not have been birthed into existence without help from the following people:

First and foremost, my Lord and Savior, Jesus Christ; He has blessed me with the talents to be able to write this book.

Secondly, to my mother, her love, acceptance, and guidance has forever changed my life and I am eternally grateful.

Finally, my awesome editor and manager, John; without him I do not think I would have a chance in Hell to get this book out into the world. His talents are a true gift from the Lord, and without them, this book would probably still be stuck in my brain, buried under everything else.

Special thanks to all of YOU for reading, supporting, and following my journey to being 'the CP Butterfly.'

May your dreams fly wild like the butterfly that God created you to be.

God bless you all!

Aleya K. Linkous

Author, CP warrior, and God's daughter.

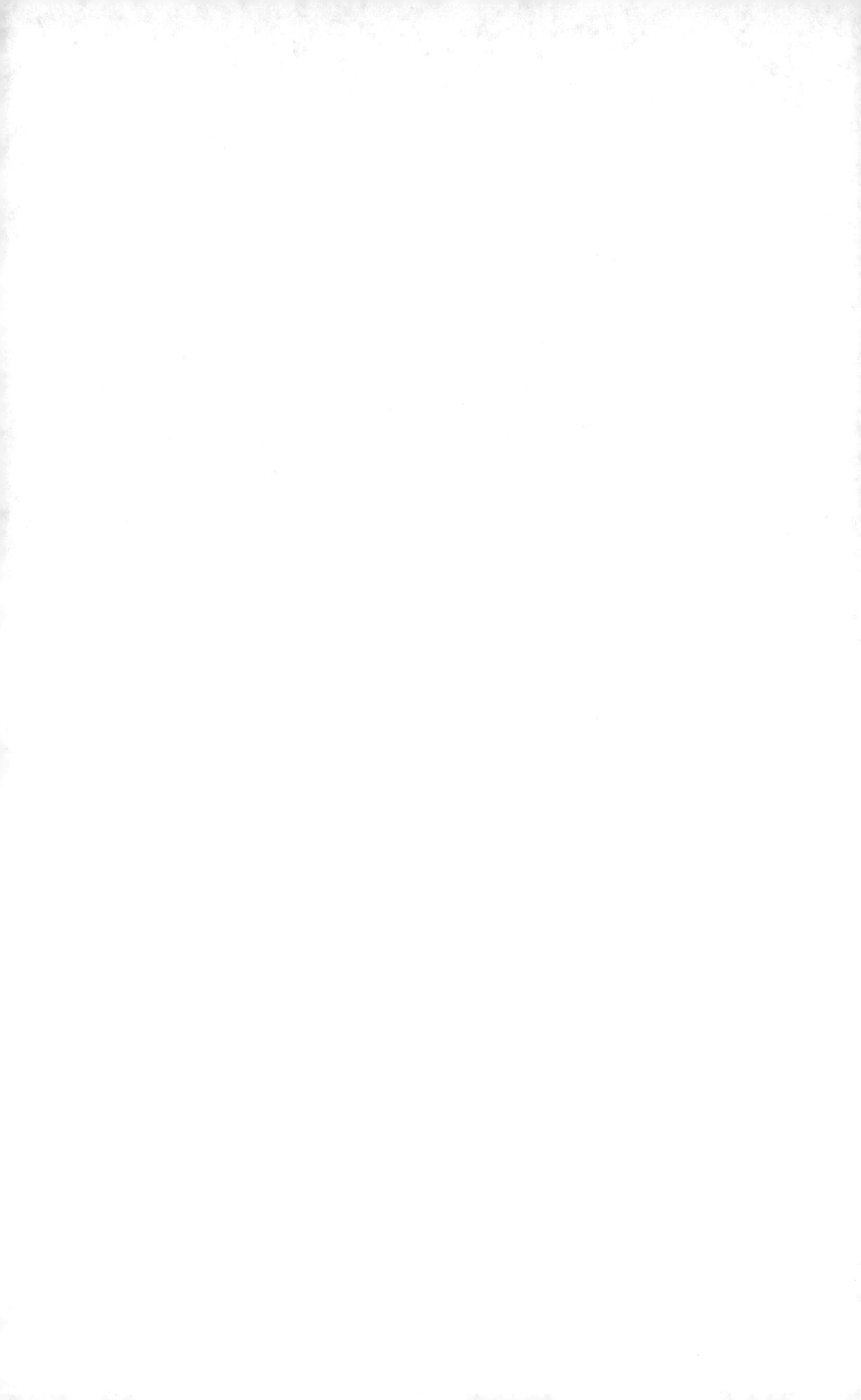

www.ingramcontent.com/pod-product-compliance
Lightning Source LLC
LaVergne TN
LVHW011051110826
845149LV00015B/3448

* 9 7 8 1 9 7 0 3 9 6 1 7 1 *